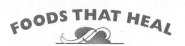

FOODS THAT HEAL

MAUREEN KENNEDY SALAMAN

THE Renew You DIET

Revolutionary New

Breakthrough Information

You'll Get

STRATFORD
PUBLISHING

IMPORTANT NOTICE

To Joel Goodrich and Sally Jordan—
two of the angels who have lifted me to my feet
when my wings had trouble remembering how to fly.

The Renew You Diet
Copyright © 2004
Maureen Kennedy Salaman

*All rights reserved. No part of this book may be reproduced in any form
or by any means without written consent of publisher/author.*

ISBN ISBN 0-913087-26-2
Third Printing

MKS, Inc.
1259 El Camino Real, Suite 1500
Menlo Park, California 94025
www.mksalaman.com
(650) 854-3922 telephone
(650) 854-5779 facsimile

Distributed by:
Maximum Living, Inc.
20071 Soulsbyville Road
Soulsbyville, California 95372-9748
www.maximizeyourlife.com
(209) 536-9300 telephone
(800) 445-4325 toll-free
(209) 536-9375 facsimile

All Scripture quotations, unless otherwise indicated, are taken from
the *King James Version*.
Literary development and interior and cover design by:
Koechel Peterson & Associates, Inc., Minneapolis, MN
Cover photo by Russ Fischella
Printed in the United States of America

CONTENTS

———— ∞∞∞ ————

Books by
Maureen Kennedy Salaman

———— ⋘∞ ————

Foods That Heal

Foods That Heal Companion Cookbook

The Diet Bible

Nutrition: The Cancer Answer II

All Your Health Questions Answered Naturally II

How to Renew You:
The Complete Primer on Age Reversal

FOODS THAT HEAL

Achieving Super Immunity

Super Heart Health

The Renew You Diet

CHAPTER ONE

RENEW YOUR MIND AND RESIST TEMPTATION

*As he thinketh in his heart,
so is he.*

—*Proverbs 23:7*

AS HE DASHED DOWN THE STEPS at Laney High School in Wilmington, North Carolina, his heart was pounding as he saw the bulletin board by the gym. There was the list that declared the names of the young men who made the basketball team. Scanning the list over and over, his name was a no-show. He had been cut from the varsity team. He wasn't good enough. He failed.

But though his dreams were crushed, he refused to give up. For the following year, come rain or shine, you could find him practicing in a park near his house for four to six hours a day. He fought through adversity and disappointment, working on every move and every shot that would help him the following season.

Michael Jordan did make the team and

became the greatest basketball player in the world. *Air Jordan* is arguably the best athlete to ever play team sports. Would he have ever achieved his greatness if he had not fought back from defeat? My guess is no.

He could have thrown in the towel and blamed his failure on the coach, but he didn't. Jordan's motto was "I can accept failure, but I cannot accept not trying." He chose a positive approach at a difficult moment and took control of his life.

YOU BECOME WHAT YOU THINK ABOUT

There is a story about a Native American boy who was talking with his grandfather. The boy asked, "Grandfather, what do you think about what's going on in the world?" The grandfather gazed back at his grandson and replied, "I feel like wolves are fighting in my heart. One is full of anger and hatred; the other is full of love, forgiveness, and peace." "So which one will win?" asked the boy. The grandfather replied, "The one I feed."

Those words echo a life-changing principle that King Solomon offered as one of his many wise proverbs, "As [a man] thinketh in his heart, so is he." How simple, yet how profound. We become what we think about. We reap the fruit of the thoughts we sow—positively or negatively.

Over a century ago, William James said, "The greatest discovery of this generation is that a human being can alter their life by altering their attitude." I believe that with all my heart, and I've seen it happen countless times during my life. I have had the joy of watching thousands of people turn their lives around through developing and maintaining a positive approach to life.

Perhaps when you picked this book up you also had the accompanying feeling that you'll never beat your weight and diet problems. One of the deepest disappointments is to set a goal, get yourself psyched up, jump into the program, and then see it collapse and fail. And repeated failure opens the door to a deluge of guilt and condemnation.

I know what that's like. I struggled with it for years. But I have good news for you. If you have failed, it just means your human. The only person who never failed is Jesus Christ. Determine right now that you will keep reading until you find the keys to success. God not only desires to help you reach your health and fitness goals, but He has a plan that will elevate you from a lifestyle of dieting to a lifestyle of freedom and self-control. He has the power to help you control what, when, and how much you eat, and He can help you get in the best shape of your life—no matter what your age.

I'm going to let you in on a secret—perhaps you've never started on the right foot in your weight-loss efforts. Perhaps your real battle begins where my battle began, and that's with a *fat mentality* that sabotages every attempt you've ever made. Putting a stake in the heart of this negative attitude is the first step to freedom.

FAT MENTALITY

"Man is the only animal who eats when he isn't hungry." Mark Twain said it, and he was right on. If you eat when you're not hungry, beware. You may have a *fat mentality*, in which you spend a disproportionate amount of time thinking and fantasizing about food. Overweight people think about food not only often but differently.

In order to trim your mind and your body, first mobilize your mentality against excess poundage through mind conditioning. Change your attitude. Recognize that more food is not necessary. Instead of unconscious eating, ask yourself, "Am I really hungry?"

You will realize you are not hungry at all. Years of conditioning through beguiling food commercials have programmed you to hone in on the refrigerator. Once you begin to withhold food, you will have hunger pangs three minutes for three days. Realize this, and let it give you some comfort. Picture in your mind those pangs helping draw your stomach tight, your thighs taut. You will win over your appetite, feel the power of enormous self-esteem, and begin to lose weight, accomplishing what you envisioned those pangs would do.

Inside of you are all the God-given capabilities needed to control your appetite, even if obesity experts tell us that some of us are programmed to be overweight. We have been given dominion over ourselves by God, so we can reprogram ourselves.

It is only hopeless if we think it is, therefore abdicating responsibility for that which your free will chooses. All it takes is sustained faith and patience to turn it around.

YEARS DO NOT EQUAL FAT

Don't blame your birthdays for your weight problem. Perhaps you have justified your weight gain by adopting the long-held belief that body fat increases naturally as people age. It's time to let go of this myth. Just because your metabolism slows down doesn't mean you're destined to gain weight.

A study published in the *Journal of the American Geriatrics Society* evaluated 679 people from 29 to 94 years old. The researchers concluded that the increased body fat often seen in older adults results from weight gain due to a sedentary lifestyle rather than an inevitable change in body composition with age. Dr. Andrew Silver, at St. Louis University School of Medicine, found no significant increase in the percentage of body fat after the age of 40. In some cultures, such as the natives of the South Sea Islands, the old are as slim as the young. They are also just as active.

Here's what does happen over time. As the hyaluronic acid in your body diminishes, collagen goes with it. You lose the underlying support scaffolding that plumps the cheeks and prevents jowls from forming. Fat in the face moves downward, creating pockets under the eyes and folds in the neck. As the skin thins, the underlying cellulite fat becomes more noticeable. The look we associate with aging is more than just added fat. It's the movement of fat. In our 20s, fat makes us look young. In our 50s, the same fat—not more of it—makes us look old. Trim the fat and build the muscle and you lose some of that aging look.

TEMPTATION

I don't like food that's too carefully arranged; it makes me think that the chef is spending too much time arranging and not enough time cooking. If I wanted a picture I'd buy a painting.

No matter what we do to our bodies, weight loss begins and ends with the mind. The first step to weight loss is eating less empty, unessential calories—those that tell our bodies to store the fat instead of burning it off. Unfortunately, calories that are of the least use to you nutritionally are the most gratifying physically. Imagine your favorite dessert; a chocolate eclair, cream puff, ice cream sundae, or my favorite—a thick, rich slice of soft, creamy tiramasu. Stop! Stop! Vacate the thought with a more positive thought!

There is a close correlation between the craving center of the brain and your eyes. Advertisers and restaurant owners know this. That's why food manufacturers spend the big bucks on professional food photographers. And why restaurants display desserts in revolving, lighted cases or on beautiful dessert carts. They know the first time you see it, you are tempted;

the second time, you are lost, and they triple dessert sales. No matter how full you are at the end of a restaurant meal, you have carried that thought over in your mind and are tempted to top it off with a sumptuous dessert. Everyone has the potential to gain too much weight.

God is faithful, who will not suffer you to be tempted above that ye are able: but will with the temptation also make a way to escape, that ye may be able to bear it (1 Corinthians 10:13).

Temptation to overeat comes in many sizes, shapes, and aromas—often so compelling that avoidance is the first line of defense. Avoidance is easier than escape, although the latter is sometimes a necessity. You know what foods turn you on and how hard it is to turn yourself off, so plot yourself a temptationless course.

Before I cover temptation, here are some of the techniques I use to avoid temptation:

1. Your first line of defense is not allowing danger foods in the house. Rid the kitchen of offending foods (you know where you store those tempting betrayers). Don't let your kids give you an excuse for buying cookies. They will thank you later.

2. Eat high bulk, low-fat snack foods between meals. Examples are Nutrition Bites (28 calories) from Maximum Living, low-fat popcorn, and apples.

3. When you eat out, don't be afraid to order an appetizer for your main course. Don't eat at

buffets, smorgasbords, or any other all-you-can-eat restaurants. It's not a coincidence that many of the people who eat at these establishments are obese.

4. Eat slowly to convince your body it is being satisfied. Chew your food 20 to 30 times per bite. Eat to slow music. Mozart wrote taffel (table) music. You'll chew in direct rhythm with the music you're listening to. You'll eat less and enjoy it more if you give your body the time to tell you that you are satisfied.

5. Divert your eyes from sweets and fatty foods in the grocery store. Don't let your eyes settle on the tempting but bad foods. And don't shop while hungry. Make a shopping list and stick to it. Bring only enough money to pay for what you need. No wandering into the middle of the store where the dead foods are. If you find yourself cruising the middle aisles, you're buying all the wrong foods. Stick to the outer aisles where the live foods are (life comes from life).

6. When you are tempted by a white or brown "unfood," visualize it as white or brown death. Then rid yourself of the thought. Don't let it take root in your mind. Replace it with the positive thought of how healthy and alive you'll look by refusing to touch it.

7. As you experience a craving, consider it a good thing and learn to enjoy it. Let denial be your friend—making you svelte, vibrant, and vigorous. Don't consider it a deprivation.

8. Listen to your stomach and stop eating when your stomach is full. You don't have to clean your plate. And if you are not hungry, don't eat. This is why most diets work at first. They make people more conscious of what they eat, how much, and if they are really hungry. Make those hunger pangs your criteria for eating.

9. The subconscious doesn't register a negative. Instead of, "No, I can't have dessert," say to yourself, "I'm too full for dessert." If you're at a dinner party, politely decline your hostess's offering while diverting your eyes from the dessert.

10. Compliment the hostess and the love and time she poured into the delicious food and eat a small portion. Don't leave uneaten portions on your plate in front of you. Call the food server or take it away from your range of vision.

11. And, most importantly, never eat after 7 p.m. I told this to a friend of mine who wanted to lose weight. When I saw him six months later I was astounded. He had lost 60 pounds! He said all he did was stop eating anything after 7 p.m. every night.

Weight loss is still a matter of eating less, exercising more, and behavioral modification. I've traveled the world and discovered cultures that eat small amounts of highly nutritious food are the people who are the healthiest and leanest, and live not only longer, but better.

While in Africa, I lived with the Masai, a joyous people who laugh easily and continuously. They eat once a day, and only as much as they are able to hold in their two cupped hands, the size of your stomach. Meals should be low fat, low calorie, and small portions. Eat dinner as early as you can or not at all. Go for a walk instead.

BELIEVE AND YE SHALL RECEIVE

Renew your mind with food substitutes: prayer, church meetings, volunteer duties, a good book, a schedule of housecleaning duties, a new hobby, a new friend, a new sport! Not only is the mind the greatest power against temptation, but you have the power to change your body from the inside out!

Practice, too, the ten-finger prayer: "I can do all things through Christ who strengthens me." Ask God for strength and the power to change. Then let His power strengthen your will.

Cover your ears. Go ahead, humor me. What you hold in your hands is the secret to a longer, healthier life. This has become such a reality to scientists that they have created a new discipline to describe it: Psychoneuroimmunology—the study of the emotion, attitudes, and beliefs of our mind as they influence the health and vitality of our body. In others words, if you think you can, you can. If you think you can't, you can't.

The next step to overcoming a "fat mentality" is to see yourself thin. God gave us a brain so we could use it. As you look in the mirror, be positive and love what you see. Imagine your waist slimmer, your hips smaller, your thighs leaner. Fully realize, in the heart God gave you, that you are worthy and deserving of what you want. Then believe it. Picture yourself the way you want to look, with sparkle in your eyes and a slim exuberance.

The best time to use positive imagery is when you are the most relaxed: before going to sleep, when waking up in the middle of the night, upon awakening in the morning. Positive imagery works from the inside out, altering your cells and body system. If you believe you will lose weight, you will.

Every time you wake up in the morning say to yourself, "I am renewing myself every day. Every day in every way I am getting better and better." Seize the day with enthusiasm. Rejoice and be glad each morning for each new day.

YOU CANNOT AFFORD THE LUXURY OF A NEGATIVE THOUGHT

In the first months of 2004, I found myself violating one my own edicts. Listening to some of the media whose treasonous tactics and lies were misleading the American people and poisoning the self-esteem of our troops in Iraq, I felt outrage and found myself caught in a web of anxiety. My three great passions are that I love God, America, and my family, and I felt the violations on all three levels. My brother is a Lieutenant Colonel in the Marines and has sacrificed so much to serve our country with honor for his whole career.

The anxiety was so intense that it finally settled over me as a depression. I expressed my anxiety for

America to my cherished friend, Dr. Fred Hudson, over dinner. And I was startled by his response. He looked me straight in the eyes and said, "Maureen, you cannot afford the luxury of a negative thought."

His words shot straight through me to the heart of the problem and set me free instantly. I couldn't allow others' negative thoughts to erode my passion and enthusiasm for life.

I cannot overstate the importance of bringing a positive attitude in your life—whether it regards weight loss or any other thing you wish to accomplish. And although I readily admit the difficulty of maintaining a positive attitude, I want you to know that it can be done. I trust that the truths you discover here will help inspire you to live your dreams.

CHAPTER TWO

FOODS THAT MAKE YOU FAT

I came from a family that considered gravy a beverage.

—Erma Bombeck

TODAY'S "CIVILIZED" AND UNNATURAL diet of man-made chemicals, hormones, and preservatives that are processed and labeled as "food" is why our nation is engrossed in an epidemic of obesity. Food preservatives, steroids injected into cattle, chemical flavorings, and artificial colorings are toxic to the body.

Evidence shows that synthetic chemicals are fattening, not in the sense of containing calories, but in damaging the body's metabolism to such a degree that weight gain occurs. While high doses of any toxic chemical will make you very sick and cause weight loss, low doses of toxic chemicals make you a little sick and a little tired, and can cause weight gain by increasing your appetite, slowing your metabolism, decreasing your ability to burn stored fat, and reducing your ability to exercise.

Sound familiar?

When the body detects chemical toxins, it protects itself by isolating those toxins so they can't damage vital organs. It does this by encasing them in fat. The more chemicals ingested, the more fat is produced by the body for protection.

HORMONES IN ANIMAL PRODUCTS

Not only is meat fattening, but the drugs in factory-farmed meat could be making people literally—if you'll forgive the expression—eat like pigs.

Let's take a look at what has happened to Shirley, who is 5'1" and weighs 325 pounds. Shirley loves meat. She loves it so much she has pounds of it delivered to her door every month, to be stored in her freezer until she cooks it for her family at every meal.

Where did Shirley's meat come from, and what happened to it before it got to her dinner table?

The farmer who raised Shirley's meat gave his steer a synthetic steroid hormone designed to cause rapid, substantial weight gain. The drug worked well. The animal became 20 percent heavier on 15 percent less food per pound than genetically similar cattle not given the drug. The steer was slaughtered with residues of the drug in his body. The drug was still working when Shirley ate it.

Shirley has consumed the residues of this drug, along with residues of other weight-promoting drugs, in her diet of beef, pork, chicken, and other meat, plus dairy products, every day for years.

Drugs that artificially stimulate the appetite were also given to the pigs, chickens, and cattle that provide Shirley's milk and meat supply, and now she has lost the ability to stop eating when her hunger has been satisfied.

How true is this to Shirley's condition: "And ye shall eat, and not be satisfied" (Leviticus 26:26).

Shirley feels hungry *all the time.* Instead of reaching the point of "can't eat another bite," she keeps going. Instead of examining what she is eating, Shirley blames her husband and the stress of raising three children. She believes her problem is emotional, not dietary. And it's killing her slowly and surely, pound after pound.

THE DANGERS OF ANIMAL PRODUCTS

Members of the European scientific community were so convinced of the dangers of hormonal beef that in 1989 they banned the import of U.S. beef into their countries. In 1998 the World Trade Organization ruled the ban illegal, citing a lack of evidence that the hormones are dangerous. Today the European Union, comprised of 15 countries, states it now has scientific evidence to justify the ban.

Unfortunately, just when the obesity epidemic is getting a lot of press, how are people trying to lose weight? By eating even more animal products, thanks to the popularity of the Atkins books, which have sold 15 million copies and are still on the bestseller list. More on the Atkins principle in chapter three, "Foods That Burn the Fat."

Over the past 20 or 30 years, as more Americans have been getting fatter, factory farmers, aided by large drug companies, have gone merrily on their way, drastically increasing the amount of antibiotics, steroids, pesticides, and other drugs they are using.

The residues of these drugs in meat, our government assures us, are so small as to be insignificant, except when some careless or greedy factory farmer continues feeding a drug until shortly before the animal is slaughtered.

A decade ago the FDA estimated that 20,000 to 30,000 different drugs were being used in food animals—90 percent of those illegally—and with testing for residues unavailable for most of them. Even assuming that it's all been straightened out now and that factory farmers are only using the 1,705 drugs officially approved by the FDA (294 of which include "weight gain" in their descriptions), there is no question that there are all kinds of drug residues in meat and dairy products. And there can be no question that these residues, over time, have become insidiously incorporated into our environment and food chain.

SUGAR MADNESS

Not surprisingly, Shirley has Type 2 diabetes. Ninety percent of people with Type 2 diabetes are obese. Type 2 diabetes occurs when glucose cannot enter body cells. Sometimes called "adult onset diabetes," it is typically diagnosed among middle-aged, overweight, inactive people.

Shirley is addicted to sugar. She thinks she doesn't eat sugar because she avoids cookies, cake, and ice cream. But what she doesn't realize is that most processed food contains large amounts of sugar in the form of corn syrup and trans-fats, which increase the body's production of sugar. It's in everything from ketchup to canned beans. One of the reasons Shirley likes the taste of processed food is because it is loaded with salt and sugar. Her taste buds have become accustomed to the sugar in her food.

Shirley thinks she is being good when she eats sugar-free candy and diet soda, buying products that contain aspartame, or NutraSweet. Aspartame is a chemical, and a potentially dangerous one at that. Better to get used to the taste of iced tea without sugar than to use the chemicals in that blue packet to sweeten it. Aspartame has been linked to diabetes, blindness, and other eye problems, brain tumors, joint pain, and even multiple sclerosis.

Shirley is not alone. Americans drink, on average, 41 gallons of soda per year. The trouble with eating refined sugar in large amounts (one can of soda qualifies) is that it stresses the body and forces the body to use up large amounts of essential B vitamins. Soft drinks contain high amounts of phosphorus as well, using up the mineral potassium. A deficiency of potassium can in turn cause a deficiency of the mineral calcium, needed for relaxed muscles and partly responsible for strong bones. Potassium is necessary for healthy skin and stable blood pressure. The B vitamin thiamine, in particular, is depleted with large amounts of sugar.

It is a vicious downward cycle that drains the body of health and vitality and opens the door to every malady. It doesn't happen overnight, but it slowly strips your body of its ability to defend itself.

Because of her poor diet, Shirley is also deficient in trace minerals. A deficiency of certain minerals has been linked to blood sugar regulation and an inability to lose weight. She is not alone here, either. A U.S. Department of Agriculture study done at Tufts University, Boston, found that 85 percent of the American public is deficient in one or more of the nutrients for which recommended daily allowances (RDAs—I call them recommended deficiency allowances) have been established. As long ago as 1936, the United States Department of Agriculture issued U.S. Senate Document 254, stating "that virtually all soils in the United States were mineral deficient." That our soils have been depleted of essential, trace, and rare minerals so vital to health is no secret.

WHAT SHIRLEY CAN DO

Shirley has to stop eating so much meat, for starters, and only meat that has no artificial growth-promoting hormones, routine antibiotics, or animal by-products. She can find that at her local health food cooperative where she can also buy organic vegetables, or start a vegetable garden. She needs to drink purified water instead of soda, and develop a taste for real food, without the salt and sugar. She needs to eat raw and fresh as much as possible.

But there is more that Shirley can do. She can increase her metabolism, overcome cravings, and regulate her blood sugar by supplementing with certain minerals. There are nutritional supplements available that can pull the toxic time bombs from her body and restore her body's natural appetite suppressant, and there are foods that will give her energy without signaling her body to store fat.

Shirley's years of poor eating have caused nutritional imbalances and deficiencies that, once eliminated, will give her the energy to incorporate exercise in her lifestyle. Her back won't hurt anymore, and her muscles will feel stronger. She'll lose the weight she needs to feel good about herself and her body.

WHAT YOU CAN DO

If a parsley farmer is sued, can they garnish his wages?

Many of today's farms use toxic chemicals on the food they produce—the food that ends up on your dinner table. How can you reduce your exposure to toxic chemicals? Since our main exposure is in foods that contain pesticides, you should go organic when possible or at least avoid the most heavily contaminated foods. Some of the same chemicals used as animal growth promoters—organophosphates and carbamates—are sprayed on foods as pesticides.

Butter is at the top of the "highly contaminated" list, with cheese and hamburger next. Heavily sprayed fruits and vegetables such as strawberries, apples, and zucchini also should be avoided unless they are organic or come from your garden. Other "highly contaminated" vegetables are leaf lettuce, kale, collard greens, broccoli, peanut butter, olive oil, peaches, and grapes. Unfortunately, most pesticide residues are systemic—they are absorbed into the plant. However, even vegetables grown organically need to be cleaned. Clean vegetables by putting them in a sink of water in which you have added a capful of hydrogen peroxide.

Eggs, meat, and dairy products can also contain antibiotics, other growth promoters, and environmental pollutants, which were not tested by the FDA. Meat and products of intensively farmed animals, such as chickens, turkeys, and pigs are also high in fattening toxic chemicals. It's well known that salmon and other fish are dangerously high in mercury. When you order fish, the grayish black layer or "mud line" that runs down the side of the fish, generally close to the lateral line, is where the toxins, including mercury and PCBs, are stored. Be sure you cut if off.

Cooking does not destroy toxic chemicals in meat and dairy products. Sometimes it makes them more toxic. Eating raw and organic as much as possible is the best way to avoid chemical additives.

If you can't live without meat, eat organically farmed, low-fat cuts of meat without the skin, because toxic chemicals and hormones accumulate in animal fat and skin. And cut down your consumption to maybe once a week.

Avoid processed foods because you don't know what was added or where the ingredients came from. Many processed foods use wheat and corn products. About 80 percent of pesticides used in America are targeted on four specific crops: corn, soybeans, cotton, and wheat, crops commonly used in animal feed as well as in processed human "food."

Now that you know what to avoid, turn the page for the next chapter on foods and supplements that help lose weight and restore health.

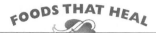

CHAPTER THREE

FOODS THAT BURN THE FAT

Feed me with the food that is needful for me.

—*Proverbs 30:8 AMP*

IF YOU COULD EAT CERTAIN FOODS you knew helped you lose weight, would you? Of course you would. A newly discovered food principle, essential to any discussion of weight loss, involves how fast or slow a particular food digests, and the amount of blood sugar—or glucose—is released as a result. I've already discussed the concept of blood sugar levels effecting weight loss. The story continues.

Carbohydrate foods that break down quickly during digestion have the highest glycemic indexes. High glycemic foods—for instance, potatoes and white bread (akin to a block of sugar)—digest quickly and pour out insulin, suppressing glycogen, which takes fat out of storage, thus increasing cravings and keeping blood sugar levels high.

As long as you are eating high glycemic foods, you are going to have trouble bringing fat out of storage. Their high sugar content creates an addiction to sugar. Because high sugar foods break down quickly, the craving is constant. As much as you desire to lose weight, you become conquered by your cravings. Let me remind you: sugar is addictive. If you ate a high sugar food in the evening for dinner, you'll want it again for breakfast or lunch. That's the trouble with addictions—they move; they never stay the same. The next morning, you'll want a doughnut.

You may believe, as many do, that we need sugar to survive. It is not denatured, processed sugar our bodies need—it is glucose, the kind of sugar that is derived from food. Even if we eat no food at all, the body will pull glucose from muscle tissue. This is why, when we fast, we lose muscle tissue as well as fat.

Can you say gluconeogenesis? This is the process the body uses to give itself energy when there is inadequate food to meet its needs for glucose. Gluconeogenesis is activated in the body when we do not eat, getting its energy by burning fat reserves. If we eat more carbohydrates than our body needs, the rest is stored in the liver and other tissues while the remainder is converted into fat.

This is why people on very strict diet plans not only lose fat, but also lose muscle tissue. Losing fat is good; losing muscle tissue is not. This is why low sugar carbohydrates—complex carbohydrates—are the foods of choice. They contain only enough glucose to energize the body and start the fat-burning process.

Complex carbohydrates break down slowly, releasing glucose gradually in the bloodstream, and have low glycemic index values. Examples are oatmeal, whole grains, and lentils. Low glycemic foods stabilize blood sugar, thereby satisfying hunger and controlling cravings, and are important to any program of weight loss.

There is a food you can accurately call a diet food. It is vinegar. As little as four teaspoons of vinegar in a vinaigrette dressing, taken with an average meal, lowers blood sugar by as much as 30 percent, plus it stimulates hydrochloric acid in the stomach, the digestive juices needed to break down food. Among the various types of vinegar, red wine is the best. Also, lemon juice has been found to be advantageous.

THE WEIGHT OF FOODS

Dr. Terry Shintani examines the weight of foods in terms of their weight-loss potential, creating a list he calls Dr. Shintani's Mass Index of Foods, or SMI. It's worth noting here because it's similar in concept to the glycemic index. The foods with the highest SMI—the highest weight per calorie—have the greatest ability to satisfy and leave us full so we don't crave more.

The average person eats between 2.6 and 4.1 pounds of food per day. Foods that rank at or above this number on the SMI will help us lose weight.

Foods highest on the SMI index—high in fiber and nutrients—include zucchini, watercress, squash, lettuce, cucumbers, celery, cabbage, asparagus, and green beans. The foods lowest are just what you would expect—bacon, beef, donuts, and cheese. Be careful using this index, however. Foods low on the SMI also include nuts and seeds, which have essential fatty acids (EFAs), important to your nervous system. For EFAs, supplement with borage oil and flaxseed oil capsules from Maximum Living.

A DANGER OF THE HIGH PROTEIN/LOW CARBOHYDRATE ATKINS DIET

One of the problems with fad diets is that people don't take the time to understand their underlying principle. They follow blindly, hoping it works. They forget that enhancing health is the goal. You don't encourage health by pigging out on fatty, hormone-laden beef and eliminating all carbohydrates from the diet. However, you do promote health and lose weight, by choosing the right forms and amounts of protein and carbohydrates.

Some people take things to extremes. If they believe a high protein diet will help them lose weight, they binge on protein foods. Meat at every meal has been a staple of the American diet since the 1950s. I believe that this common practice is one of the reasons we suffer from cancer, Alzheimer's and heart disease, and age-related diseases such as cataracts and strokes. Now we know why.

Free-floating enzymes are used to digest protein. Too much protein in the diet and these enzymes become used up and unavailable to the body. When we get enough enzymes to digest protein and still have enough to patrol the body, they are free-floating. They enter the bloodstream and become potent anti-inflammatories. When they are missing, the body's natural inflammatory immune response—when cells swell to discharge sickness—fails to check the inflammation, and it becomes chronic.

Since the 1970s, I have been saying that chronic inflammation is to blame for many of our life-threatening diseases, and that enzymes are the solution to this inflammation problem.

Now, conventional science has finally heard me. The cover of *Time* magazine for February 23, 2004, was titled: "The Secret Killer: The surprising link between INFLAMMATION and HEART ATTACKS, ALZHEIMER'S, CANCER, and other diseases." Hardly a week goes by without the publication of yet another study uncovering a new way that chronic inflammation does harm to the body. It destabilizes cholesterol deposits in the coronary arteries, leading to heart attacks and strokes. It chews up nerve cells in the brains of Alzheimer's victims. It even encourages the mutation of cells into cancer. In other words, chronic inflammation may be the engine that drives many of the most feared illnesses of middle and old age.

If you are eating a lot of protein, or have a

family history of heart disease, circulation problems, strokes, Alzheimer's, and cancer, take digestive enzymes with your meals in a supplement such as Multi-Enzyme. It helps with absorption and digestion of your foods. Include the free-floating enzyme formula Enzyme Ease. Enzyme Ease is coated so the enzymes move through your stomach and are released into the bloodstream—free-floating—where they can prevent the chronic inflammation that causes cancer and other diseases.

Read my award-winning book, *Nutrition: The Cancer Answer II*, if you are interested in learning more about this. It was voted the best health book in the U.S. and has won awards in Great Britain, Australia, and the Philippines. There is a whole chapter on enzymes, and it is still the best information out there.

Maximum Living's Enzyme Ease also supports the digestive organs. Pancreatin is an enzyme used by the pancreas to digest fats. When there are inadequate pancreatic enzymes, fat goes where it shouldn't—your thighs, butt, and belly. When enzymes are absorbed into the bloodstream instead of the stomach, they also prevent the inflammation and swelling that contributes to weight gain. Enzymes that enter the bloodstream also help detoxify the body, turning off the body's alarm system that forms fat to protect itself against chemical toxins.

If you are following the Atkins diet, there is one more reason to supplement with enzymes.

The Atkins diet forbids too many of the best fruits. The fruits highest in sugar/carbohydrates are the ones highest in enzymes. Examples are pineapple and papaya.

LOWERING CARBOHYDRATE INTAKE SAFELY

Lowering carbohydrate intake means eating less of the high glycemic foods, those that contain starch and sugar. These include the obvious— white bread, white rice, potatoes in any form, pasta, candy, baked goodies, ice cream, chips, and soda pop. Not so obvious are most deli-style meats, meat loaves, ham, corned beef, bacon, and sausage, which have sugar and/or starch filler added. Many canned fish products have sugar and/or starch-added sauces. All types of dairy products have some carbs—cheese, cream cheese, sour cream, and yogurt. Beware of the "light" and "low-fat" types of dairy products; these definitely have starches used as fillers.

Be careful that, if you choose the Atkins diet, you don't go overboard on restricting carbohydrates. Low-carb regimens such as the Atkins and South Beach diets restrict the intake of certain fruits, vegetables, and grains, therefore shorting the vitamins and minerals strategic to your good health, good looks, and good function. Whole grains contain B vitamins and vitamin E, vital to the brain and good mental health.

Besides robbing the body of key nutrients, low-carb eating plans can also impact thinking ability. When a body is robbed of carbohydrates, it draws its energy from ketones, a byproduct that results from breaking down body fat.

This process explains some of the dramatic weight loss that can be achieved with eating plans that restrict carbohydrate intake. But ketones have a dulling effect on the brain. Low-carb diets work by fooling the body into thinking that it's starving. This quasi-starvation mode is not good for alertness, memory, or thinking.

Carbohydrate loading is used by endurance athletes for a good reason—it gives their bodies an extra storage of fuel so their performance increases dramatically. Restricting carbohydrates endangers your energy, endurance, and performance in your work, your workouts, and in everyday life.

Rather than restricting carbohydrates, choose the best ones wisely and let them help you lose weight.

BURNING FAT WITH APPETITE-CONTROLLING CARBOHYDRATES

Complex carbohydrates such as brown rice, beans, lentils, or whole grain bread not only are digested slowly, thus stabilizing blood sugar, but their high fiber content helps control the appetite and increase energy.

Carbohydrates have been getting a lot of bad press lately. But what they don't tell you is the difference between the good and the bad. Simple carbohydrates, such as bread, potatoes, and white rice, are high glycemic and induce the body to store fat, which is bad. Complex carbohydrates, such as what I'm describing here, help the body burn fat. That's good.

Do you crave sweets in the morning and fats for lunch? Make a habit of eating complex carbohydrate foods such as lentils, kidney, navy, or pinto beans for breakfast. For lunch, have a salad with vinegar and olive oil and maybe some whole grain bread drizzled with olive oil. Make sure that whatever food you eat, it is whole, raw, and contains its natural fiber.

Beans are great for weight loss and regulating blood sugar because their natural sugars are burned off slowly, thereby stabilizing blood glucose and acting as an appetite suppressant. Beans also contain B vitamins, which are important to the nervous system, brain function, and energy level.

SOY—A HEALTHY SOURCE OF CARBOHYDRATES *AND* PROTEIN

There is a natural, nutritionally complete meal replacement product I am very excited about. I love the taste and smooth, chewy consistency. It's called "Maximum Living Nutrition Bites, the feel-full snack." It nourishes muscle, helps burn the fat, and restores the body to optimum health. I've tried it, and it works for me. It is packaged as chewy nuggets and comes in three flavors: chocolate, vanilla nut, and peanut butter.

Its main ingredient is organic soy protein, a

healthy, easily digested protein that helps convert fat into muscle. The soy protein in these tasty snacks also contains many other vital nutrients, including fat-reducing enzymes, nitrogen, and amino acids. And this soy is "non GMO," meaning it is certified as non-genetically modified or manipulated.

Centuries of making people both healthy and slim have proven what a health-giving food soy is. Derived from soybeans, it is rich in soluble and insoluble fiber and contains the good fats (monounsaturated and polyunsaturated) as well as both omega-3 and omega-6 fatty acids, which help the body move out the bad lumpy fat while at the same time moisturizing the skin from the inside out. Not only does soy contain no cholesterol, but it is also known for its ability to reduce cholesterol levels. Soy also contains all eight of the essential amino acids not manufactured by the body, and isoflavonoids, which act as natural non-steroidal estrogen. Soybeans, a known cancer fighter, are eaten in great quantities in Japan and China, and is one of the reasons researchers believe these countries have low rates of breast cancer and few menopausal symptoms.

Maximum Living Nutrition Bites have all of the good stuff and none of the bad stuff. They have all the nutrients necessary to lose weight and build lean muscle: essential fatty acids, amino acids, minerals, and soy protein. Unlike most products like it, they contain no hydrogenated oils or refined sugar. The following fat-burning ingredients are in them: biotin, because it helps eliminate the body's need for glucose, increasing the body's ability to burn fat and reversing the unhealthy aspects of being overweight; chromium for blood sugar regulation, an important factor in weight loss; lecithin and the minerals zinc and copper, so as the pounds roll off, your skin will stay tight, firm, and beautiful; and digestive enzymes that speed up weight loss by encouraging thorough digestion so nothing is left to be stored as fat.

PROTEIN TO BUILD MUSCLE

Later I'll cover the importance of exercise to build muscle and burn fat. Protein is essential to build muscle. If you are going to eat animal protein, be sure the animals are range-fed and antibiotic- and hormone-free. Protein is also found in vegetables. Vegetable protein contains many vital nutrients, including fat-reducing enzymes, nitrogen, and amino acids.

The argument made by the egg and meat people in favor of their products has been that vegetables have incomplete protein—that is, there isn't one kind that contains all the essential amino acids. All foods contain some amount of protein. In order to get complete protein in one meal, you simply have to know how to combine them properly.

To reach your daily allowance of complete protein combine whole grains with legumes. For example, the Greek dish felafel combines whole wheat pita bread with garbanzo beans. It happens to be a healthy, fast, finger food, not to mention a delicious meal. Latin Americans get their protein by combining corn tortillas with beans. In India it's rice or wheat chapatis with lentils. Since cooking destroys many essential amino acids and vital digestive enzymes, avoid processed foods and eat your veggies raw.

Other protein plant food combinations are nuts and seeds with legumes, and nuts and seeds with dark green leafy vegetables. Eat a green salad with kidney beans and sunflower seeds. There you have it: a good source of protein and lots of other essential nutrients!

FAT-BUSTING FIBER

One of the many missing or deficient ingredients in today's foods is fiber. Numerous studies have found that the average daily diet contains only 15 grams of fiber, roughly half of the National Cancer Institute's recommended 25 to 30 grams. A fiber conspicuous by its absence in processed foods is bran.

Fiber is one of the best dietary aids for weight loss or control, because it moves food quickly through the digestive system, slows down the absorption of simple carbohydrates, and delays the feeling of hunger. It contains very few calories and offers a great deal of bowel bulk. Perhaps fiber is most welcome in your dietary plan because it gives you the feeling of being full, decreasing the temptation to overeat. Even before that, fibrous vegetables and fruits demand chewing, which in turn increases the amount of saliva and reduces food intake.

When fiber is mentioned, most people think in terms of bran—wheat, rye, oat, or rice. But the range of fibers breaks out beyond the grains spectrum into beans, lentils, vegetables, and fruit. While wheat bran rates highest in fiber content, blackberries, dried prunes, and apples with skin are excellent. Of course, vegetables such as celery and carrots and asparagus are high glycemic, too.

Psyllium and hyssop are two excellent fibers that help aid in weight loss. Psyllium, known for its cholesterol-lowering properties, and hyssop, valued as an excellent source of fiber, is contained in Maximum Living's Hyssop Cleanse.

David, of the Bible, knew the benefits of hyssop. He drew lessons from the remedy, which he used in showing cleansing, for he said, "Purge me with hyssop, and I shall be clean; wash me, and I shall be whiter than snow" (Psalm 51:7).

DIGEST FAT WITH ENZYMES

With improved digestion and absorption, the body stores less fat. In order to achieve optimal digestion, and therefore fat assimilation, enzymes are essential. Digestive enzymes help the body re-absorb fat that has gone where it doesn't belong. If you don't get enough of these enzymes from vegetables and fruit, you risk gaining weight.

There are two ways of taking enzymes— three, if you count eating fruits and vegetables.

But for the best therapeutic effect, target supplemental enzymes.

The best formula for helping digest food and fat is Maximum Living's Multi-Enzyme, which contain all natural enzymes necessary to ensure everything goes where it is supposed to. For maximum health and potency, these are grown and harvested from organic, one-quarter seed sprouts rather than synthetic chemicals that barely mimic plant enzymes.

Especially if you are implementing a low-carb, high-protein diet, you need to be aware of the need for the digestive enzymes that thoroughly break down protein, carbohydrates (whole grains), and fats. These are amylase, protease, and lipase. They function as biological catalysts, making sure that all the food you eat is used and properly distributed. If your food isn't digested, the body stores it as fat.

To ensure your food is used for energy, and not stored as fat, supplement every meal with Maximum Living's Multi-Enzyme. The tablets are designed to dissolve rapidly in the stomach and Betaine HCl is included to ensure adequate stomach acid so food is broken down efficiently.

Take Multi-Enzyme with every meal. I carry a small plastic bag of enzymes with me so that I have them for every meal. If I eat protein for dinner, I take 6 to 8 tablets. Add Hyssop Cleanse for faster weight loss. I saw one woman lose a dress size the first time she tried this combination.

AMINO ACIDS STOKE THE FIRE

In this booklet I will discuss how exercise causes the body to burn fat. Amino acids mimic this effect. They work like this:

Our trillions of cells have mitochondria, minuscule furnaces in which fats and carbohydrates are burned, changing into energy. This burning calorie effect is called thermogenesis. Fat has difficulty penetrating the inner sanctum of the mitochondria, where the action is. Amino acids join hands with fat and move it into the mitochondria for burning.

If the body is low in amino acids, delivery of fat into the mitochondria will be slow, leaving surplus fat to accumulate. Carnitine, one of the amino acids, makes body fat burn faster; a low level does just the opposite. The human body can synthesize carnitine from the amino acid lysine, with a little help from its friend the amino acid methionine. Men are more richly endowed with carnitine than women, which theoretically should make them able to burn fat faster. Obviously, you need all the amino acids together for optimum benefit.

Amino acids are like the slats of a barrel. You need the full set, and one is only as effective as the shortest slat. For full supplemental benefit, look for a formula that includes all the free-form amino acids, such as Maximum Living's amino acid formula, which is all natural and derived from a hypoallergenic whey source. The amino acids contained in this formula are naturally sourced, so they contain natural tryptophan, the precursor of serotonin, which satisfies hunger and is a natural mood elevator.

BROWN FAT

Fat burning fat? Yes, it is possible. We have something in our bodies called "brown fat." It is the 10 to 20 percent of total body fat that is located deep in the body and is bound to the skeleton. This fat generates heat to regulate body temperature and, when working at full steam, helps burn off the bad fat, closest to the skin. Brown fat explains how hibernating bears keep warm yet lose weight while they sleep.

When excess calories are consumed, brown fat compensates in part by producing more heat to burn off the calories instead of storing them as white fat. The amount of brown fat in the body and its activity explains why some people can overeat and stay slim while other people gain weight easily. Brown fat becomes less active, and less able to burn, with age. Therefore, keeping brown fat activated is a big key to weight control. Brown fat activity goes down with a lack of exercise and nutrient deficiencies.

Gamma Linolenic Acid (GLA), also known as omega-6, is an essential fatty acid contained in greatest amounts in borage oil which, I know, sounds like something you put in the crankcase of your car. It comes from the blue star flower and has been shown to not only activate brown fat cells, but may increase calorie burning and decrease storage of white fat. Essential fatty acids are polyunsaturated fats, the kind of fats we need for good health and fat distribution. Obese people typically have less polyunsaturated fat in their bodies than thin people. I take Maximum Living borage oil and I don't have to starve myself to remain thin.

Omega-6 fats are hard to come by in today's modern diet as its food sources are not commonly eaten in adequate amounts. When was the last time you ate raw nuts or seeds? The wild birds in your backyard are likely eating better than you are. When was the last time you saw an obese bird? We eat nuts and seeds that have been roasted, the omega-6 cooked out of them. Some raw vegetables have omega-6 oils until they are processed for a long shelf life. Omega-6 oils go rancid quickly, which is why processed foods don't contain them, and why supplemental formulas are best.

Important to realize also, is that a lack of vitamins, minerals, and, most important, essential fatty acids reduces the efficiency of brown fat function. Always supplement with complete vitamin and mineral formulas.

The heat-producing factory of brown fat is stimulated through meals of complex carbohydrates, moderate protein, and low fat, but exercise remains the most effective way to get the kind of action you want out of your distribution of brown fat.

Later I'll show you how exercise can stoke the fires burning calories and fat, while increasing muscle mass, necessary to keep those home fires burning.

CHAPTER FOUR

CAUSES (AND SOLUTIONS) OF WEIGHT GAIN

> *Lucy decided to forget her weight just this once and enjoy herself. This was a decision she made with deplorable frequency.*
>
> —Josephine Tey

MANY WEIGHT-LOSS PROGRAMS don't work because they don't identify and eliminate the cause. Granted, eating too much food and usually the wrong foods are the main causes of weight gain, which is where most of the emphasis in weight loss is placed. All food contains potential energy, which is defined as "calories." When we eat food, either we use the food and burn it up as energy, or it gets stored on our body as fat. If we keep eating more food than we burn, we get fat.

But when you look in the mirror and lament your love handles, spare tire, or saddlebags, consider the possibility that the source might be far different than you've ever imagined.

WATER WEIGHT OR FAT GAIN?

Did you ever consider that you're looking at water weight gain rather than fat gain? Just as your nose and chest become congested in order to wash out germs and cold viruses, the body swells with water, also known as edema or dropsy, in order to defend itself from perceived foreign particles.

But where does the water come from, and why is it there? One reason is toxic buildup. It's not a coincidence that in an environment of unprecedented chemical outgassing from automobiles, carpets, and plastics, our society at the same time experiences unprecedented obesity. Your immune system is constantly defending itself from the effects of the Industrial Revolution.

Other reasons the body retains water are an imbalance of minerals and food allergies. But for now, I'll talk about the toxins.

The typical human fat cell has 50 and 100 chemical toxins. Why are toxins in fat cells? Because the body stores them there to keep them out of the bloodstream and away from vital organs. It's the only place they can go without causing harm. The body also attempts to dilute them by engorging the fat cells with water. The more toxins, the more fat and water is produced. In the unending circle of life everything goes some place. That's why fat goes on the butt, hips, thigh, and stomach. The body actually manufactures fat to house and store toxins to keep them from vital organs. It's operating for your survival in spite of yourself.

From where do we get these toxins? Medications, drugs, alcohol, cigarettes, pesticides, food additives, air, water, chemical pollutants, and fat-adding hormones injected into cattle and chicken, and the milk, butter, and eggs that come from them. Even our own body produces toxins, such as when you are fighting an infection or allergy.

The Environmental Protection Agency (EPA) estimates that there are about a half a billion chemicals in use today. And every year we add 5,000 new ones. Up to 25 percent of these chemicals have been shown in studies to cause cancer. There have been relatively few studies done on these chemicals combined. Remember, we are not just getting that one toxin they are studying and emphasizing—we are getting thousands of them combined, and we are getting bombarded with them. So that is the reason you hear a lot lately about detoxification. Detoxification is extremely important to getting and maintaining a sleek and healthy body.

One of the newest discoveries related to detoxification is the benefits of glutathione—an antioxidant amino acid. Glutathione deals directly with fat-soluble toxins—those that accumulate in body fat—such as pesticides, heavy metals and solvents. It works by allowing them to be diluted in water— making them water soluble—so the kidneys can safely eliminate them. High levels of glutathione are found in the lungs, where it corrals the toxins in smoke, smog, and other airborne pollutants. But it is particularly concentrated in the liver, your body's primary organ for detoxification.

To get your daily diet of glutathione, eat foods rich in it. They include raw fruits and vegetables such as avocado, broccoli, kale, and cauliflower. Cooking destroys the amino acid.

If you don't eat as well as you know you should, Maximum Living's antioxidant formula contains excellent levels of glutathione and vitamin C, which increases blood levels of glutathione. It also includes cysteine, which helps boost its detoxifying effect.

Another way to detoxify is through a good fiber supplement that pulls toxic time bombs out of the intestines before they can influence the immune system. Maximum Living's Hyssop Cleanse uses hyssop with psyllium, the best source of fiber available. It also includes detoxifying herbals such as goldenseal, alfalfa, and oat bran. m-u Boost, another Maximum Living product, is especially designed to boost the immune system's ability to render toxins harmless.

Antioxidants with good quality essential fatty acids, such as borage oil and flaxseed oil, activate lipids (the fat turnover) and the toxic chemicals that sit in the adipose tissue and the nerve cells. If you do this about three times a week, you can remove approximately 66 percent of the toxic chemicals in your body in around four weeks' time. According to Hans Kugler, Ph.D., one of the world's leading authorities on health and aging, you can also expect to lose unwanted weight in the process of eliminating the chemicals.

FOOD ALLERGIES

If your weight fluctuates, especially if you feel heavier at the end of the day, consider the possibility that you have food allergies. Food allergies can cause water retention and, thus, weight. When the body reacts to an allergen, it swells to minimize the effect. If, when you wake up in the morning, your tongue has small tooth-shaped wedges grooved into the side of it, chances are you have food allergies. There is a simple, scientific test you can perform to identify your food allergens in my book *All Your Health Questions Answered Naturally*.

Identifying and eliminating food allergens can stop this cycle. Common food allergens are dairy, beef, sugar, chocolate, eggs, citrus fruits, coffee, corn, malt, pork, potatoes, tomatoes, wheat, and yeast.

Nutritionally, vitamin C with bioflavonoids can help retard the inflammatory effect of food allergies since bioflavonoids, particularly quercetin, are natural anti-inflammatories. Quercetin and other bioflavonoids are included in Maximum Living's Solu-C products.

To ensure the breakdown of food and to encourage full digestion, take a full-force enzyme formula. Remember in my book, *How to Renew You*, I explained that one of the ways nature ages us is to cut back our ability to absorb and digest our nutrients. Maximum Living's Multi-Enzyme has everything you need to digest your food, and for systemic benefit, choose Enzyme Ease, which is coated so enzymes pass through the stomach, are absorbed into the bloodstream and digest necrotic tissue toxins. These enzyme products are superior to others because they are derived from live, 1/4-inch seed sprouts, the most potent source of nutrients in vegetables—grown, sprouted and harvested under the most meticulous conditions.

MINERAL DEFICIENCIES

The meek shall inherit the earth, but not the mineral rights.

One way you can tell if you have mineral deficiencies is if your ankles and legs swell. Without adequate minerals, the body retains sodium and water, which can be overcome by increasing your intake of minerals and vitamin B12. Sodium works in concert with potassium and other minerals. Minerals also help the body compensate for increased fluid caused by allergies and toxins.

More than 99 percent of the U.S. population is deficient in trace minerals, according to U.S. Government document #249. According to U.S. Senate document #264, our farm and range soils have been depleted of nutritional minerals with the result being that crops grown on these soils are mineral-deficient.

A deficiency of certain minerals has been linked to those ups and downs in our blood sugar that cause our resolve to be conquered by our cravings, making it hard to lose weight. They include chromium, a mineral used to treat low blood sugar. Chromium reduces insulin resistance, which in turn decreases our storage of body fat and increases its metabolism. Since chromium helps stabilize blood sugar levels, it also may reduce the feeling of hunger.

Vanadium, a little-known mineral, works with chromium and is important in regulating blood sugar. It stabilizes cholesterol levels, helping to prevent circulation blockages. Because of its glucose-regulating qualities, it can help battle fatigue, depression, and nervous exhaustion. It is found in safflower, olive, and sunflower oils, whole grains, herring, sardines, and liver.

These minerals are vitally important to your health, yet dangerously rare in the modern diet. They are more likely to be in short supply than other minerals, and are, perhaps, the missing link in the incredible epidemic of obese and overweight Americans.

I protect myself by taking a mineral in solution formula, which includes vitamin B12 and the optimum ratio of one to three of calcium to magnesium. It's called MineralRich, and I highly recommend it.

HYPOTHYROIDISM

An inability to lose weight can also be caused by an under-functioning thyroid, called hypothyroidism. Although it weighs only a mere two-thirds of an ounce, the thyroid gland is the largest gland in the neck and is phenomenally important to your overall health. Your thyroid gland makes, stores, and releases the thyroid hormone directly into your bloodstream for delivery to your cells wherever and whenever it is needed. When the thyroid is under-functioning, which happens in hundreds of thousands of people, and especially women, the metabolism slows and it can become difficult to lose weight.

The late Broda O. Barnes, M.D., Ph.D., was a world-renowned thyroid authority. He concluded that first generation hypothyroids often can correct their condition by taking a kelp tablet daily. Kelp is rich in iodine, the thyroid's major nutrient. Hypothyroids of the second generation or beyond can overcome depression and many other symptoms of low thyroid function by taking a natural, desiccated thyroid supplement. I recommend Armor Thyroid. Unlike synthetic thyroid hormone, Armor is natural and has no long term side effects.

To get Armor, you can contact Rodrigo Rodriguez, M.D., at the International Bio Care Hospital & Medical Center. Call 18007850490. You can have a doctor visit on the phone, and he will prescribe and mail it to you. The total cost will be about $30.

Iodine is so thoroughly deficient in our natural foods that it had to be added to salt to avoid epidemics of goiter. Adding iodine to table salt began in Michigan, where in 1924 the goiter rate was an incredible 47 percent. Iodine deficiency is now rare in the United States.

When choosing a mineral formula, look for one that contains iodine with other minerals derived from natural sources. MineralRich contains iodine and all the nutrients necessary to avoid any mineral deficiency.

Dr. Barnes' best contribution toward public awareness of thyroid problems was in all likelihood the Barnes Basal Temperature Test. This is a simple test that can be done by anyone in the privacy of his own home.

Since your body temperature reflects your metabolic rate (which is largely determined by hormones secreted by the thyroid gland), the state of the gland can be determined by taking your temperature. All that is needed is a thermometer.

Shake down the thermometer and place it by your bed before going to sleep. When you wake up, prior to getting out of bed, place the thermometer under your armpit for a full ten minutes. Stay as still as possible. After ten minutes, read and record the temperature and the date. Record the temperature for at least three consecutive mornings, preferably at the same time. Menstruating women should perform the test on the second, third, and fourth days of menstruation.

Your body temperature should be between 97.6°F and 98.2°F. Anything lower is indicative of hypothyroidism; anything higher may indicate hyperthyroidism.

HORMONES

Hormones are a major problem when it comes

to weight loss. For two years, I've been working with two women on their weight. While they have both adjusted their eating habits, neither has lost fat. I recently discovered that both are taking synthetic hormones. Believe it or not, as much as 35 pounds of their weight is a side effect of the hormones.

The connection between hormones, especially synthetic, is actually very simple. The female body needs equal amounts of progesterone and estrogen. Over time, females produce less progesterone and estrogen, but the progesterone is lost at a lower rate, causing an imbalance.

There is a strong connection between fat and estrogen. Next to the ovaries, fat is the most significant source of estrogen in the body. Women can get caught up in a cycle where increased body fat raises estrogen levels, and estrogen increases a tendency to accumulate body fat.

As if this weren't bad enough, fat cells under the influence of estrogen are "greedier" than other fat cells. Estrogen-affected fat cells tend to hold on to fat more stringently, and release it more grudgingly than cells not impacted by estrogen. The fat cells most influenced by estrogen are found predominantly in the hips, thighs, and buttocks. I can relate!

Women gain an average of 10 to 15 pounds at menopause, and, as if the fat issue wasn't enough, estrogen also promotes water retention. When synthetic hormones replace natural hormones, this estrogen dominance becomes more pronounced. Even men have estrogen dominance because of their daily exposure to 7.1 billion pounds of estrogen-mimicking pesticides and the synthetic estrogens used to fatten cattle, pigs, and chickens, and to increase milk production. More about this issue in the chapter, "Foods That Make You Fat."

What can you do about it? You can gradually, and naturally, restore your levels of progesterone. You do this by supplementing with natural progesterone cream, which is absorbed into the skin and is taken up by the fatty layer beneath. It is then transferred into the bloodstream, where it circulates to progesterone receptor sites throughout the body. In the case of the aforementioned hypothyroid issue, progesterone will make thyroid hormone receptors more sensitive and, thus, aid thyroid activity in the body.

Maximum Living's ProgestiMax topical progesterone cream includes pregnenolone and DHEA (dehydroepiandrosterone), which have connections to the adrenals and have proven advantageous to menopausal women and older men. DHEA is an androgen, one of the hormones reduced during menopause.

Maximum Living's Vita-Sprout is a non-synthetic multi-vitamin formula that is high in B complex vitamins from organic vegetable sprouts (the most potent form of nutrients possible). It balances iodine with zinc, selenium, and potassium, B vitamins for the nervous system, and other nutrients. The B vitamins choline and inositol in Vita-Sprout help the liver break down estrogen into estriol, a non-carcinogenic form of the hormone (estradiol is the carcinogenic form). B vitamins also can reduce many of the symptoms of premenstrual syndrome.

YEAST INFECTIONS

Candida Albicans, or yeast infection, has been associated with weight gain, and is often caused by chronic use of antibiotics. It can be fought with supplemental beneficial bacteria, e.g.: lacto-bacillus acidophilus, which is found in yogurt and other cultured food, and in Hyssop Cleanse.

CRASH DIETS

At first crash diets seem to work. Then they begin to work you over. Intemperately low-calorie food intake triggers the body's set point—your obstinate archenemy against losing weight, a built-in biochemical mechanisms that protects the body against starvation and a survival system that automatically lowers the metabolic rate, the rate at which food is burned in the cells.

You are wonderfully made—all of the 60 to 70 trillion cells that are you. And these cells raise a subliminal fuss when they sense that you're not feeding them enough, particularly when you're on a crash diet or skipping meals! However, with God's adaptability created in you, you have meta-bolic machinery that slows down when you're on a diet, and especially when it's a drastic one.

Here's what typically happens. You cut your caloric intake to 900 calories, and then your body slows its metabolism to compensate. You tire of the Spartan torture and eventually go back to your normal caloric intake—say, 2,000 calories. Now your body's thermostat has been set to burn up 900 calories. So you have a surplus of 1,100 calories over what your metabolism is geared to handle. Where do those calories go? To all the old familiar places as fat. Sure, the metabolism eventually comes into balance and burns faster and hotter, but first you gain back all the fat you lost in your martyrdom and more.

But the damage can't be measured solely in terms of calories. If you pursued a regular exercise program along with the low-cal diet, you undoubtedly lost more than just fat: you lost some muscle and protein tissue. You came out of this with a poor exchange. You lost fat, muscle, and other protein, and you gained back fat only—that is, unless you continued your exercise.

Research has shown that people who continue to gain and lose weight find it ever more difficult to lose weight. Yo-yo dieting makes a person use food less efficiently and increases the difficulty in subsequent dieting efforts.

To outwit this compensatory mechanism, don't decrease your caloric intake radically. A 600- to 800-calorie diet will only serve to jangle all the alarm bells, whereas a gradual decrease in food intake will not as readily let the set point know what's going on. The secret is to eat less, stop the empty calorie foods such as sugar and white flour, exercise more, and stay with a solid program for the rest of your life.

STOMACH REDUCTION SURGERY— A LAST RESORT FOR OBESITY

Stanley James Rogers, M.D., Assistant Professor of Surgery with the Bariatric Surgery Center, UCSF, tells me the number-one surgery he performs is bariatric (obesity) surgery that reduces the size of the stomach so obese individuals, whose weight is jeopardizing their health, can lose a large amount of their excess weight. Patients will not necessarily be "thin" as a result of these operations, but their excess weight will typically decrease by about two-thirds within two years. Dr. John P. Cello, Professor of Medicine and Surgery, UCSF, concurs. They are the Top Guns of this surgical specialty, and I was honored to talk with them.

Bariatric surgery should only be considered as a last resort to life-threatening obesity. Obesity is defined as having a Body Mass Index (BMI) of 40+ or being at least 100 pounds overweight.

Gastric bypass surgery is the most common procedure, but not the only one. In Gastric bypass, the stomach is stapled so that it has the capacity of 2 to 3 ounces. Then a piece of small intestine is attached to the new stomach so that food passes to the small intestine. The stomach is so small that when only 2 to 3 ounces of food enters, hunger is quickly stopped.

The other procedures are too numerous and complicated to go into here. Suffice it to say, the extent by which the stomach is reduced can be varied and even adjustable, using bands positioned differently around the stomach, closing it off. The advantage of bands is that they are adjustable and even removable.

Americans will put up with anything provided it doesn't block traffic. Surgery is not an easy answer to weight loss. It certainly isn't the answer to weight loss. I'm sorry to disappoint you, but after consulting with Dr. Rogers, I learned that even if you choose this route, if you don't change the way you eat you will gain the weight back again. Surgery is a difficult battle but it doesn't win the war.

CHAPTER FIVE

BURN THE FAT WITH EXERCISE (the Atom Bomb of Your Weight-Loss Arsenal)

Food fuels the furnace of metabolism; exercise stokes its fire.

—Majid Ali, M.D.

ONCE YOU HAVE ACCOMPLISHED ALL THAT I have recommended in the preceding chapters, you should have the energy and ability to do what will help you lose weight the fastest: EXERCISE. This word deserves tall capital letters, it is that important.

The experts agree: burning calories loses weight faster and more efficiently than reducing calories. Stanford researchers discovered that women who did not exercise and ate 300 calories less than their caloric requirements actually gained more weight than avid tennis players who ate 600 calories more than their daily requirements. Adding exercise to a moderate diet almost doubles the percent of body fat loss.

How much is enough? Experts recommend that you do a half hour of moderate aerobic activity at least three times a week for instant calorie burning, plus weight-bearing exercise to convert fat into muscle and keep your metabolism primed.

I love skiing. To me, there is no experience of freedom quite like flying down a ski hill.

The Bible gives little attention to exercise, undoubtedly because when men from Abraham to Jesus needed to get from here to there, they walked fifteen to twenty miles a day and thought nothing of it. They performed every sort of manual labor. Ninety-five percent of their work was physical. Now only about five percent of typical work is physical.

FEEL THE BURN TO STOKE THE FURNACE

The more you exercise, the more energy you have and the happier you feel. This is due to the endorphins that are released when you exercise. Ask a marathon runner about the feel-good endorphins released by the brain during physical exercise. Endorphins are happy hormones hundreds of times more powerful than the strongest morphine. Endorphins create a natural "high" that is a mood elevator. Endorphins reduce stress, improve mood, increase circulation, and relieve pain. The more you exercise, the more endorphins you release.

Endorphins stoke the fire of your mitochondria, the power plant or furnace of the cell that produces energy. During exercise the mitochondria creates many more mitochondria. Because of this expansion, you have more energy during exercise. Mitochondria generally come out of the liver at a rate of 30 to 40 per hour. When we exercise, they come out at a rate of 300 to 400 per hour. More exercise means more muscle on your body and less fat.

Do you want to burn fat? Do you want to lose body fat, increase your strength and energy, and produce visible improvements in muscle tone within weeks? Start working out! When you increase muscle, you rev your metabolism—then watch the pounds melt off!

You've heard the term "feel the burn"? Exercise instructors use it to describe the burning sensation resulting from strenuous exercise. It's also an indicator that thermogenesis is at work—burning white fat in the furnace of your body.

Regular, spirited exercise will burn off surplus fat better than moderate exercise. Studies reveal that dynamic, big-muscle exercises such as running and bicycling generate metabolic (fat-burning) rates that are eight to ten times higher than what you burn when resting. Vigorous physical activity can continue to burn fat up to fifteen hours after exercise.

IF VIGOROUS IS PAINFUL,
TRY SUSTAINED EXERCISE

The word aerobics comes from two Greek words: aero, meaning "ability to," and bics, meaning "withstand tremendous boredom" (Dave Barry).

You don't have to bounce and bobble your way to a good figure. Rather, you can experience burn by lifting your leg repeatedly. This simple exercise will burn fat and build muscle.

Vigorous exercise burns fat faster than moderate exercise, but moderate exercise still burns fat. Any fat-burning exercise merely requires slow, sustained activity.

Want to feel the burn without jumping jacks? Try this. Hold your arm out, palm upward. Now lift it up. Do it twice. No problem, right? Now, do it twenty times. Did you feel the burn? Now do it while holding a can of soup. Better yet, hold my book, *All Your Health Questions Answered Naturally*. You just increased the burn by including something heavy. This is called weight- or resistance-training.

If you are careful not to overdo it, stretch thoroughly before any workout, including walking, and take it a little at a time, increasing repetitions instead of weight, you shouldn't have a lot of pain when you exercise.

Start a daily routine of walking a block or two, then increase gradually. Walking exercises all your internal organs. If you want to get rid of that spare tire around your waist, start jumping rope for 22 minutes a day. Moderate, daily exercise protects from disease. As you walk to exercise your legs and lower body, carry weights and swing your arms to burn off the fat in your arms and upper body. Weight-bearing exercise prevents osteoporosis and increases strength, agility, and health, even in the most fragile. It truly is never too late when it comes to exercise.

You can burn fat while watching TV. From your couch or chair, lift your legs twenty times. Next add ankle weights. Now you're doing weight-training. This form of exercise not only burns fat but increases muscle. If you keep adding weight, you'll keep adding muscle (more so for men, but women can do it too). As you gradually add weight (or resistance), you add strength. If you keep it up, you can compete with body-builders. And it doesn't matter how old you are— even if you're 95 you can do it!

As I mentioned before, building muscle through regular strength training enables you to burn more calories every single day—even while you are resting. One pound of muscle burns 35 to 50 calories a day. Compare that to a paltry two calories burned by a pound of fat!

Orchestra conductors have notoriously strong arms and cardiovascular health because of the repetitive motion their profession requires. Swimming is good for burning fat because of the resistance provided by water. Most classes begin with water exercises (to increase stamina) before getting out there to sprint and tread water for 30 minutes at a time. For the less ambitious, water aerobics offers resistance with less work, and it's great for cardiovascular fitness.

BEST TIME TO EXERCISE

When is the best time of day to do aerobic exercise? The answer is any time! The most important thing is that you just do it. Continuous cardiovascular exercise, such as walking, jogging, stair climbing, or cycling, sustained for at least 30 minutes, will burn body fat no matter when you do it.

However, if you want to get the maximum benefits possible from every minute you invest in your workouts, then you should consider getting up early and exercising before you eat breakfast—even if you're not a "morning person." Early morning aerobic exercise on an empty stomach has three major advantages over exercising later in the day:

Early in the morning before you eat, your levels of stored carbohydrates are low. What you want to do when you exercise is burn fat, not carbohydrates. This is best accomplished on an empty stomach. Some studies have suggested that up to 300 percent more fat is burned when you exercise on an empty stomach. Carbohydrates (glycogen) is your body's primary and preferred energy source. When your primary fuel source is in short supply, this forces your body to tap into its secondary or reserve energy source—body fat.

If you exercise immediately after eating a meal, you'll still burn fat, but you'll burn less of it because you'll be burning off the carbohydrates you ate first.

The second benefit you'll get from early morning exercise sessions is what I call the "afterburn" effect. When you exercise in the morning, you not only burn fat during the session, but you also continue to burn fat at an accelerated rate after the workout. Why? Because an intense session of cardiovascular exercise can keep your metabolism elevated for hours after the session is over. If you exercise at night, you will still burn fat during the session, so you definitely benefit from it. However, it fails to take advantage of the "afterburn" effect because your metabolism drops like a ton of bricks as soon as you go to sleep. While you sleep, your metabolic rate is slower than any other time of the day.

Burning more fat isn't the only reason you should do your exercise early. The third benefit of morning workouts is the endorphine "rush" and feeling of accomplishment that stays with you all day long after an invigorating workout.

Exercise can be a pleasant and enjoyable experience, but the more difficult or challenging it is for you, the more important it is to get it out of the way early. When you put off any task you consider unpleasant, it hangs over you all day long, leaving you with a feeling of guilt, stress, and incompleteness (not to mention that you are more likely to "blow off" an evening workout if you are tired from a long day at work or if your pals try to persuade you to join them for dinner).

MAKE WEIGHT LOSS A LIFESTYLE CHOICE

Pound for pound, muscle burns five times as many calories as other body tissues. The addition of ten pounds of muscle to the body can burn 600 calories more a day. That means after the first three months or so, you can cut down and take it easy without seeing the pounds come back. Here are some ways in which you can burn calories without trying—very hard.

1. Make it a habit of stretching before you retire at night and after you get up in the morning. Pull your arms over your head, stretch them from side to side, and flex your legs and feet. Stretch before doing any form of strenuous exercise, including a brisk walk to the park or store. Feel the burn as you stretch? You're burning calories!

2. Chew on crushed ice instead of snacks. Oklahoma City physician Charlie Farr says that when you lower your temperature by eating ice, your body raises its metabolism (the rate at which your body burns calories). By drinking eight 16-ounce glasses (one gallon) of purified, unchemicalized ice water a day, you can burn up to 300 calories.

3. Eat barley bread, which is high in the mineral chromium. Barley contains almost six micrograms of chromium per gram of grain. Studies have shown that chromium helps the body lose fat and make muscle.

4. Instead of the elevator, take the stairs—two at a time. A day's total of 15 minutes will put you

more than 220 calories ahead.

5. If you take the bus or subway to work, walk to the next stop or get off a stop or two early and hoof the rest of the distance. At work, get up every hour and cruise the floor. Walk to a coworker's office instead of phoning.

6. Instead of going out, take a walk for lunch, then pick up some deli on the way back. Walk to the restaurant. A mile of brisk walking five days a week burns up the caloric equivalent of seven pounds of fat in a year!

7. Instead of plopping in front of the TV or going to the movies over the weekend, spend free time with the family in active, calorie-burning fun. Thirty minutes of bowling burns 200 calories (or go alone and bowl three games in a row), an hour of Ping-Pong can burn 300 calories, and 20 minutes of skating will burn off 200 calories.

8. Park in the very last spot and walk briskly to the store or to work.

9. Clean the gutters (lose 100 calories in 16 minutes).

10. Rake the leaves or rake the grass. Does your lawn need aerating?

11. Plant a tree. Volunteer to plant a tree.

12. Paint your house. It's not as hard as you might think.

13. Push-mow the lawn. Today's reel mowers are not like you remember. Thanks to technology that has improved the design, it has become the Stairmaster of the 1990s. The American Lawn

Mower Company—one of only two reel mower manufacturers in the country—sold about 100,000 mowers in 1990, an 80 percent increase over 1988 sales. In general, pushing a mower will burn 275 to 350 calories an hour, which puts it on a par with recreational tennis and moderate cycling. You might even call it a mild form of cross training, since it can tone up several large muscle groups, depending on your technique.

14. Wash the car every week. Wax it every month.

15. Play with your kids. An hour of play can burn between 250 to 300 calories. Be an airplane. Lie on the floor face up. Holding your child's hands, place your feet, knees bent, on the child's stomach. Push upward until the child's torso is balanced on your feet. Keep your knees slightly bent. Holding hands, you can lower and raise the child, giving your legs a hefty workout. The child can hold his/her arms outward, mocking an airplane's wings, while balancing on your feet. Play dodge ball, basketball, or hopscotch.

16. Cut and stack firewood.

17. Keep a weekly list of household chores and do them. Your house will be cleaner, and you'll be fitter. An hour of scrubbing can burn up to 300 calories. Ironing for an hour will burn slightly more than 100 calories; 30 minutes of mopping the floor yields about the same.

18. Give your husband/wife a full body massage.

19. Crush cans for recycling.

20. Volunteer to pick up trash along the highway.

21. Clean houses for extra money. It's a lot more interesting when it's someone else's house.

22. Clean construction sites for extra money. Check with a temporary work agency and you won't be committing yourself for long-term duty. If you like to do woodwork, you can pick up good quality scrap lumber for nothing.

23. Plan a month ahead, picking different activities every week. Give yourself exercise options that you can look forward to.

24. Join an exercise club or group that meet once or twice a week. Exercising with others is much more fun than going it alone.

25. Don't use a scale. Muscle weighs more than fat. Go by how you feel and how your clothes fit instead.

Never give up. Never accept defeat. And whatever you do, do it regularly. If you make exercise part of your lifestyle, you'll feel good in your body for the rest of your life.

CHAPTER SIX

MAUREEN'S TEN STEPS TO WEIGHT LOSS

But I keep under my body, and bring it into subjection...

—1 Corinthians 9:27

WHILE THERE ARE A THOUSAND "do's" and "don'ts" for weight loss, I'm going to give you 10 practical steps that I assure you will renew you and bring you closer to where you want to be. I know that in doing the "do's," many "don'ts" will automatically take care of themselves. It is far more effective to keep your focus on what you should do instead of always reminding yourself of what you shouldn't.

While you may struggle with the idea of exercise and changing your diet, keep in mind that how you feel about it is far less important than how it will make you feel and look. On the days when you exercise and eat right, you will feel better all day long. And that good feeling is going to propel you into a new lifestyle that will give you the health and fitness you've been dreaming about.

You have the power to renew you, so start today!

1. Exercise every day. Walk one day, take an aerobic class the next, lift weights the next. Take dance classes. Take lessons. Skip rope. Learn how to play racquetball, golf, or dance. Vary your exercise to keep you interested. My personal trainer, Charles Wright, makes certain that my exercise routine is different every day so that I continue to work different muscle groups and that I don't get bored. It works wonders!

2. Increase your production of the human growth hormone (HGH) by guarding your sleep as well as by exercising. HGH helps keep us slim, builds bone density, and converts fat into muscle. But HGH diminishes as we get older, and greater care must be given to its production. Studies have shown that when we increase human growth hormone through a variety of ways, we lose fat.

The best and most reliable way to get HGH is to increase your output naturally. The first way to do this is by not eating before bed. Why? Because the process of digestion is the heaviest energy demand on the body and interferes with deep sleep, and HGH increases during the deepest part of sleep, REM sleep, when you dream. Don't eat for two, ideally three, hours before bedtime. Bedtime snacks suppress the release and fat-burning effects of HGH.

You also need to commit yourself to eight hours of sleep. Realize that your body responds to artificial light, which confuses it into thinking it should be alert even though it is dark outside. You should dim the lights for 45 minutes before going to bed and take two SweetSleep melatonin capsules from Maximum Living. Melatonin is a hormone that promotes sleep and contributes to the circadian rhythm—the sleep-wake rhythm—and body temperature. We have exhausted it with electric bright lights at night, extending our days and exhausting our youthifying melatonin. SweetSleep will aid your natural melatonin and give your REM the restorative power God meant it to have.

Intense physical exercise also increases the production of HGH. So not only does a good workout help you build muscle, but it helps reverse aging.

3. Eat no sugar and no more than two servings of fruit a day. Eliminate high-sugar (high-carbohydrate) fruits such as mango, peaches, and bananas. Target low-carb apples, grapes, and watermelon. For sugar withdrawal, eat Maximum Living Nutrition Bites (described in chapter three). They are sweetened by melted brown rice with just a smidgen of honey.

4. Avoid processed grains. This means white bread, white or instant rice, and dry pasta. All your grains should be whole, not processed. Limit your bread consumption to whole grains and only two pieces a day. Be sparing with butter.

5. Eat protein food only at breakfast or lunch. Have lentils, kidney beans, navy beans, or pinto beans for breakfast. For dinner, have a salad. Buy organic.

6. To keep the body's fat-burning oven stoked continuously, for between-meal snacks eat lean

foods or two Maximum Living Nutrition Bites nuggets. Target foods such as apples, celery sticks, and cauliflower. Eat an apple a day, chewed slowly with a large glass of water. A chocolate Nutrition Bite with an apple is delicious, healthy, and slimming.

7. Eat no dairy products, including cheese, for the first three weeks. Because weight gain is associated with food allergies, and because dairy products are common allergens, staying off dairy products for a few weeks might tell you how much they are to blame.

8. Supplement with MineralRich. Among other benefits, it contains a 3-to-1 ratio of magnesium to calcium in solution, which will not only encourage weight loss but help reverse aging. When you are born, your cells are 95 percent magnesium and five percent calcium. Under a microscope they are translucent. When you die of arterial disease, your cells are 95 percent calcium and only five percent magnesium. MineralRich contains chromium, vanadium, and biotin for craving control. You'll notice you experience cravings during certain times of the day. Pay attention to when your cravings occur, and take MineralRich half an hour before they happen. It will stabilize your blood sugar, the underlying cause of your cravings.

Also supplement with borage oil, flaxseed oil, enzymes, vitamin E, Vita-Sprout, Nutrition Bites, Hyssop Cleanse, and amino acids. Together they will keep cravings—and weight—under control.

9. When dining out, if there are portions left

on the plate, leave or have the plate taken away. Don't keep looking at it. There is a very close relationship between the craving center of the brain and the eyes. The first time you see it, you are tempted. The second time you are lost. Vacate the thought from your mind once you have seen it. Remember, your stomach is the size of your two hands cupped together. Try to limit your intake to the amount your hands will hold.

10. Drink lots and lots of water. Drink at least eight 16-ounce glasses. Nothing makes you lose excess fluid like drinking a lot of water, so it's good for losing water weight.

Remember, you didn't put on those extra pounds overnight. Therefore, you must realize that those pounds are not going to come off in a couple of days. You must have patience, perseverance, be disciplined, and understand that to lose the weight and keep it off you must be willing to make permanent changes in your approach to eating and exercise.

Most importantly, never lose sight of your goal, and remember that good health and longevity are your primary objectives.

Remember, God rewards faithfulness. The fact that you, as well as your family, friends, and business associates, may consider you more attractive and you will have a more energetic and confident approach to life are tremendous, but merely "secondary" benefits. Vibrant health is its own reward.

Malcolm Forbes said it best, "Diamonds are just chunks of coal that stuck with it."

MAUREEN SALAMAN continues to formulate leading-edge products based on the latest scientific research and highest production standards to ensure the natural force and power of the nutrients are retained. This expertise and her leadership are a vital part of the Maximum Living company.

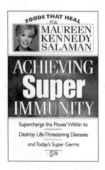

Also in this Series

#610 / $7.95

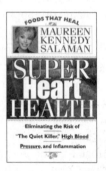

Also in this Series

#625 / $7.95

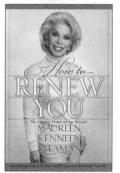
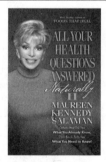
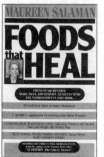

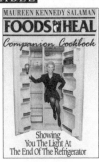
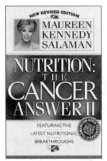
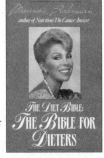